CH00665373

Save Your Life with Stupendous Spices

Becoming pH Balanced in an Unbalanced World

by

Blythe Ayne, Ph.D.

Books by Blythe Ayne, Ph.D.

Nonfiction:
Love Is The Answer
45 Ways To Excellent Life
Horn of Plenty—The Cornucopia of Your Life

How to Save Your Life Series:
Save Your Life With The Power Of pH Balance
Save Your Life With The Phenomenal Lemon
Save Your Life with Stupendous Spices
Save Your Life with the Elixir of Water

Fiction:
The Darling Undesirables Series:
The Heart of Leo - short story prequel
The Darling Undesirables
Moons Rising
The Inventor's Clone
Heart's Quest

Short Story Collections:
5 Minute Stories
13 Lovely Frights for Lonely Nights

Children's Illustrated Books:
The Rat Who Didn't Like Rats
The Rat Who Didn't Like Christmas

Poetry & Photography:
Life Flows on the River of Love
Home & the Surrounding Territory

Audio:
The Power of pH Balance –
Dr. Blythe Ayne Interviews Steven Acuff

Save Your Life with Stupendous Spices

Becoming pH Balanced in an Unbalanced World

by

Blythe Ayne, Ph.D.

Save Your Life with Stupendous Spices
Blythe Ayne

Emerson & Tilman, Publishers
129 Pendleton Way #55
Washougal, WA 98671

Book & cover design by Blythe Ayne
All Text & Graphics © 2017 Blythe Ayne

Save Your Life with Stupendous Spices

www.BlytheAyne.com

Paperback ISBN: 978-1-947151-08-6
Hardback ISBN: 978-1-947151-28-4
ebook ISBN: 978-1-947151-09-3

[1. HEALTH & FITNESS / Diet & Nutrition / Nutrition
2. HEALTH & FITNESS / Healing
3. HEA049000 HEALTH & FITNESS / Longevity

BIC: FM

First Edition

Table of Contents

Introduction

Save Your Life with Stupendous Spices

Gold? Frankincense? Myrrh? No – *even better!* Turmeric, Ginger, Cinnamon, and Sea Salt.

In ***Save Your Life with Stupendous Spices*** you'll read a few of the astounding benefits these four Gifts of Earth have to offer – truly the ***Spice of Life!***

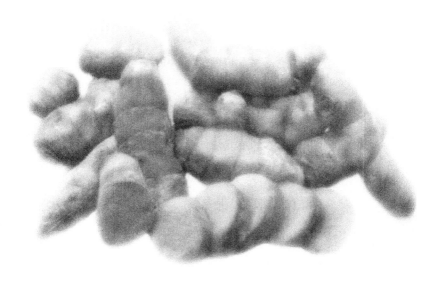

Turmeric

Turmeric, which is related to ginger, is the bright yellow spice commonly found in curry powder. It's one of nature's most powerful healers, and has a long history of human use for both internal and external use.

Under intense and ongoing research, its medicinal properties are the subject of over 5,600 biomedical studies, resulting in over 600 potential preventive and therapeutic applications, and 175 distinct, beneficial, physiological effects.

Turmeric root is actually a rhizome – is a continuously growing horizontal underground stem that puts out lateral shoots, rather than roots. *Curcumin*, the active ingredient in turmeric, is an antioxidant compound found in the rhizome of the turmeric plant, and is more effective than vitamin E. The rhizomes of turmeric enhance immune function by stimulating white blood cells. Curcumin also protects DNA strands from breakage.

Known for its anti-inflammatory, antiseptic, antibacterial, and antimicrobial properties, research has revealed that turmeric is beneficial in the treatment of numerous health conditions, even very serious ones, including cancers and Alzheimer's.

An interesting fact is that India has the highest per capita consumption of turmeric, and the lowest incidence of cognitive decline worldwide – coincidence? I think not!

Turmeric's Numerous Benefits
Check out this "short list" of but a few of the benefits of turmeric's curcumin:

Turmeric boosts cognitive function by binding to and dissolving the dangerous beta-amyloid protein plaque in the brain, that contributes significantly to cognitive decline in people with Alzheimer's disease.

It supports muscle and joint strength, and helps the body respond appropriately to inflammatory aches and pains. It's a powerful anti-inflammatory that works as well as many anti-inflammatory drugs, *without the negative side effects*. It's a natural anti-inflammatory treatment for arthritis and rheumatoid arthritis.

A man was diagnosed with a severe inflammatory disease of the joints and was heavily medicated with high-priced drugs that didn't help. He reports that he found turmeric root in his local supermarket and started chewing the root in one-inch pieces, and claims that every single one of his symptoms vanished in two days.

This same response of curcumin to aches and pains also contributes to excellent heart health. Curcumin protects against cardiovascular disease with its mild anti-thrombotic process, and it inhibits platelets from clumping together.

Curcumin works with the function of the liver, providing healthy detoxification.

It works fantastically as an anti-inflammatory agent for the treatment of digestive problems.

Turmeric aids in fat metabolism and assists with healthy weight loss. These beneficial effects were demonstrated in a study of two groups of obese mice. The group without turmeric developed diabetes. The group with turmeric showed diabetic symptoms diminish, *and even disappear!*

Turmeric is a natural painkiller and is a cox-2 inhibitor. Cox-2 (cyclooxygenase-2), is an enzyme responsible for inflammation and pain. Turmeric is an effective treatment for inflammation of the mouth.

Here are a few more personal reports regarding the positive effect of turmeric for various health issues:

"I had a painful cyst on my wrist. My friend suggested taking turmeric capsules. The cyst went away in a week!"

"When I don't take two teaspoons of turmeric every day, my bursitis pain and inflammation in my shoulders returns."

"I'm 78 and still employed as a nurse. I do a lot of walking. I've been taking turmeric for 3 years, I have no pain and I sleep like a baby. Before starting to take turmeric, my arthritis was painful and made me stiff."

"I had a bad sinus infection that had been with me for weeks and nothing seemed to help. A friend told me about the turmeric health drink and my infection was cured within 3 days."

In addition to all the foregoing, turmeric is a natural mood enhancer, having been used for many years as a treatment for depression in Chinese medicine.

Turmeric in Research

And here are but a few of the effects of turmeric's curcumin on various cancers in the numerous, ongoing studies:

First and foremost, turmeric appears to prevent metastases from occurring in many forms of cancer, and has anti-mutagenic activity.

Research has thus far shown that turmeric can suppress the development of stomach, breast, colon, lung, and skin tumors.

Turmeric has been shown to cause melanoma cells to self-destruct, and may even *prevent* melanoma.

Curcumin prevented breast cancer from spreading to the lungs in mice.

Curcumin appears to stop the growth of existing prostate cancer when combined with cauliflower, and again, may *prevent* prostate cancer from the outset.

Studies show positive effects of turmeric on inhibiting multiple myeloma.

It has been shown to stop the growth of new blood vessels in tumors.

Turmeric augments the positive effects of the chemotherapy drug paclitaxel and reduces its side effects.

There is evidence that turmeric slows the progression of multiple sclerosis in mice.

It reduces the risk of childhood leukemia.

But it doesn't only work on the inside! Curcumin contributes to beautiful, healthy, radiant skin, keeping it glowing and smooth. It has proven helpful in the treatment of psoriasis.

It's an antiseptic and antibacterial that speeds up wound healing and assists in repairing damaged skin. Applied topically it quickly clears up insect bites, poison ivy, cuts, burns and other inflammatory skin conditions, and heals an eye infection if used in a compress.

Turmeric is recommended for people who suffer from gall stones, *though with caution!* The good news is that curcumin stimulates the release of bile from the gall bladder and can assist in the reduction and release of gall stones over time. The bad news is, if this healing action is too sudden, forceful or energetic, it can cause the opposite to occur.

Please undertake a regime of turmeric and/or ginger to heal your gall bladder under the supervision of your naturopathic or homeopathic health care provider.

An Ounce of Prevention

The benefit of turmeric is in its rhizome. You can often find turmeric rhizomes near the ginger rhizomes in health food stores and many grocery stores. I like to get the little "fingers" of turmeric, and munch one of them down, raw, as a rule, one a day. It's a bit like a carrot, but stronger. It has a nice, crunchy texture. This is a great way to get the whole goodness turmeric has to offer.

Of course, it's great grated into your foods. I have a little grater that's perfect for the little rhizomes of turmeric. I get these little rhizomes because, I've learned, if I grate from a larger section of turmeric and put it back in the refrigerator, it tends to go bad before long. Whereas the skin-enclosed little rhizomes stay good for much longer.

You can also get a tincture of turmeric, which is very good. Keep it on the kitchen counter and squeeze half a dropper into body-temperature water and drink it down, to make sure you have your daily dose.

Turmeric also comes in capsule form, and, of course, as a spice in powdered form, used in cooking.

For health benefits, it's recommended to have two teaspoons of turmeric a day. Also, because the beneficial aspects of spices are not entirely bioavailable, it's a good idea to take turmeric with piperine. Piperine is the alkaloid in black pepper that produces pepper's aroma, flavor, and health benefits—which also increases the bioavailability of nutrients in foods, supplements and spices.

Barring the availability of peperine, fresh ground black pepper, and also cayenne pepper, contribute to releasing turmeric's golden treasures.

Supercalifragilistic Health Drink
2 tsp. turmeric
1 lemon (either the juice, or, if blending, using the entire lemon – *excellent!*)
1 tablespoon honey
Piperine (if available)
Cayenne pepper to taste
1 cup of water

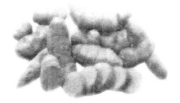

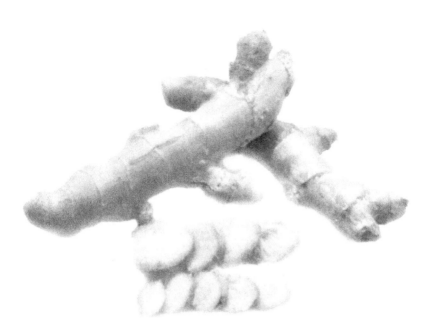

Ginger

Beautifully aromatic, ginger, with its powerful anti-inflammatory, anti-fungal, anti-ulcer, anti-tumor, antioxidant, antibacterial, and pain-relieving properties has been a health remedy for ailments, aches, pains and diseases for centuries.

Native to Southeastern Asia, ginger is mentioned in ancient Chinese, Indian, and Middle Eastern writings, appreciated for its culinary and medicinal uses.

At the same time, its piquant, spicy flavor adds zest to fruit and vegetable dishes alike. The really good news is that it's readily available and affordable in your local market, all year long.

Current researchers are discovering that ginger works wonders in the treatment of a wide range of disorders and diseases, from migraines to cancer.

The ginger root – actually a rhizome like turmeric, has an outer skin and an interior firm flesh. The health benefits of ginger come from *gingerols* and *shogaol* – Ginger's active phytonutrients, powerful anti-inflammatory compounds.

Ginger as a Natural Remedy
Happy Tummy!
Ginger is probably most commonly known as being very effective in relieving stomach upset, and is also used to stimulate appetite.

It's used to treat chronic indigestion and dyspepsia, which is caused by delayed emptying of the stomach during a meal. Ginger has been shown to speed up the emptying of the stomach, and is also effective in alleviating colic.

Many studies have proven that ginger prevents the symptoms of motion sickness, even more effectively than Dramamine. It reduces *all* symptoms of motion sickness, including nausea, dizziness, cold sweats and throwing up.

It is equally effective with morning sickness, including the most severe forms which require hospitalization. In addition to reducing the severity and number of morning sickness attacks, it's also extremely safe – unlike drugs prescribed for this condition, which *can cause birth defects!* It only takes a small amount of ginger to provide relief.

Ginger is also helpful in reducing water retention, healing stomach flu, and treating food poisoning.

Ginger in Your Home Arsenal

Ginger has proven to be a significant weapon in the treatment of numerous ailments and diseases. Let's look at a few more of the many ways it can be used in your day to day life as a natural curative.

The antioxidants and bioactive compounds in ginger inhibit inflammatory responses in the brain, including Alzheimer's and Parkinson's diseases.

Ginger provides relief from migraine headache due to its ability to stop prostaglandins from causing pain and inflammation of the blood vessels in the brain, which leads to migraines. Ginger is also an effective treatment for earache.

Because of its antibacterial and anti-fungal properties, ginger can be used for reducing toothache and the discomfort of an infection in the upper respiratory tract.

Another common cause of respiratory infections is the RSV virus, which fresh ginger is effective in treating.

Ginger has long been used as a treatment for colds and the flu as a natural decongestant and antihistamine. It is also an excellent treatment for shortness of breath and asthma.

It is very effective against inflammatory diseases of the gum, the bacteria gingivitis and periodontitis.

Ginger in the form of tea is a natural heartburn remedy.

Ginger is also used in the treatment of external wounds, including snake bite.

Ginger boosts bone health and relieves joint pains. It produces marked relief in arthritis pain.

Ginger is strongly recommended for people who have diabetes, as well as people who suffer from heart problems. Ginger lowers cholesterol, while boosting the pumping action of heart.

Ginger is recommended for people who suffer from gall stones, though with the same caution as noted under turmeric. Ginger stimulates the release of bile from the gall bladder and can assist in the reduction and release of gall stones over time, but if the healing action is too sudden or energetic, it can cause inflammation and blockage.

Please undertake a regime of turmeric and/or ginger to heal your gall bladder under the supervision of your naturopathic or homeopathic health care provider.

Ginger is an effective treatment for exercise-induced muscle pain. Though it appears not to have an immediate impact, it reduces the day-to-day progression of muscle pain.

Ginger in Research

Let's take a look at some of the research with ginger....

Research has discovered that ginger has an effect on blood clots similar to aspirin.

Brain Function

Oxidative stress and chronic inflammation accelerate the aging process, believed to be among the key drivers of Alzheimer's disease and age-related cognitive decline. There are numerous studies with animals showing that ginger protects against age-related decline in brain function, enhancing brain function directly.

In a study of sixty middle-aged women, ginger extract was shown to improve reaction time and working memory.

Cancers

Ginger's phytonutrients, gingerols, induced cell death in all ovarian cancer cells by inducing apoptosis – programmed cell death, and autophagocytosis – self-digestion, in Studies at the University of Michigan Comprehensive Cancer Center.

Inflammation is believed to be central to the development of ovarian cancer. In the presence of ginger, a number of key indicators of inflammation, interleukin-8 and prostaglandin E2, were decreased in the ovarian cancer cells.

Although conventional chemotherapeutic drugs initially suppress inflammatory markers, it appears that cancer cells eventually become resistant to drugs. But ovarian cancer cells exposed to ginger *do not become resistant to its cancer-destroying effects.*

A study at the University of Minnesota found that ginger may slow the growth of colorectal cancer cells. The results with a study of mice with colorectal cancer injected with gingerol were so significant that the researchers went on record saying that the ginger compounds are effective chemopreventive and chemotherapeutic agents for the treatment of colorectal carcinomas.

Diabetes

A study on diabetic rats found that rats given ginger had a reduced incidence of diabetic kidney damage known as nephropathy.

In a recent study, forty-one participants with type 2 diabetes took two grams of ginger powder per day, resulting in a 12 percent reduction in fasting blood sugar.

It also dramatically improved HbA1c, a marker for long-term blood sugar levels, with a 10 percent reduction over a period of twelve weeks.

There was a 23 percent reduction in markers for oxidized lipoproteins, and a 28 percent reduction in the ApoB/ApoA-I ratio. Both are major risk factors for heart disease.

Osteoarthritis & Rheumatoid Arthritis
Arthritis is a degeneration of the joints in the body, leading to severe joint pain and stiffness.

Gingerols are playing a major role in the lives of people with osteoarthritis or rheumatoid arthritis. The significance of the reduction in their pain levels and improvements in their mobility when they consume ginger regularly is quite reassuring. In two clinical studies physicians found that 75 percent of their patients with arthritis experienced relief of pain and/or swelling.

In another study over a period of twelve months, 29 patients with painful arthritis in the knee participated in a placebo-controlled, double-blind, crossover study. Patients switched from placebo to ginger or visa versa after three months.

By the end of six months, participants given ginger were experiencing significantly less pain than those given a placebo. Pain decreased from a score of 76.14 to 41.00. Those who were switched from ginger to placebo experienced an increase in pain, up to 82.10.

In the final phase of the study all patients received ginger. Pain remained low in those already taking ginger in phase 2, and decreased again in the group that had been on placebo.

In addition to the pain reduction of ginger, the objective measurement of swelling in the knees dropped significantly! The knee circumference in those taking ginger dropped from 43.25 cm when the study began to 39.36 cm by the twelfth week.

When this group was switched to placebo in the second phase of the study, their knee circumferences increased, while those who had been on placebo were now switched to ginger experienced a decrease in knee circumference. In the final phase, when both groups were given ginger, knee circumference continued to drop.

An investigation of how ginger works was the subject of a study on gingerol, where it was shown to significantly inhibit the production of nitric oxide, a highly reactive nitrogen molecule that forms peroxynitrite, a damaging free radical.

In other research, ginger has been shown to suppress the inflammatory compounds cytokines and chemokines, produced by synoviocytes – cells comprising the synovial lining of the joints, chrondrocytes – cells comprising joint cartilage, and leukocytes – immune cells.

In a controlled trial of 247 people with osteoarthritis of the knee, everyone who took ginger extract had less pain and required less pain medication.

Cholesterol
High levels of LDL lipoproteins – the harmful cholesterol – are linked to an increased risk of heart disease.

Three grams of ginger powder daily, in a 45-day study of 85 people with high cholesterol, caused significant reduction in cholesterol and excessive triglycerides.

Ginger extract was as effective as the drug atorvastatin in lowering LDL cholesterol in a study of hypothyroid rats.

An Ounce of Prevention
You can enjoy the rhizome of ginger fresh, powdered, dried as a spice, as an oil, or as juice. Ginger is also available crystallized, candied, and pickled. *Yum!*

Keep ginger powder in a tightly sealed glass container in a cool, dark, dry place, or in the refrigerator where it will have an extended shelf life of about one year.

Fresh ginger can be stored in the refrigerator for up to three weeks if it is left un-peeled. Stored un-peeled in the freezer, it will keep for up to six months.

Choose fresh ginger over dried – it's not only superior in flavor but contains higher levels of gingerol as well as ginger's active protease, the enzyme that breaks down proteins and peptides, and that provides anti-inflammatory action.

Make sure the ginger root your buy is firm, smooth, and free of mold. Organic is best, of course, and it's important to get ginger (or any spice!) that has not been irradiated. Irradiated produce is given 35,000 more radiation than that allowed for x-rays, and kills off the good with the supposed bad.

One-third teaspoon of powdered ginger taken at the outset of a migraine will help stop the pain before it has had its way.

For nausea, ginger tea made by steeping one or two 1/2-inch slices of fresh ginger in a cup of hot water will settle your stomach.

For arthritis, some people have found relief in as little as a 1/4-inch slice of fresh ginger cooked in food, although more is better and quicker.

In a study of 30 individuals, two grams of ginger extract per day significantly reduced inflammatory signaling molecules in the colon.

Ginger lemonade is delicious! Combine freshly grated ginger, lemon juice, honey and water.

Grated ginger is *great* on just about any dish from roasted vegetables to ice cream to a bowl of fruit.

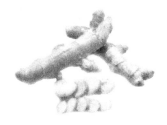

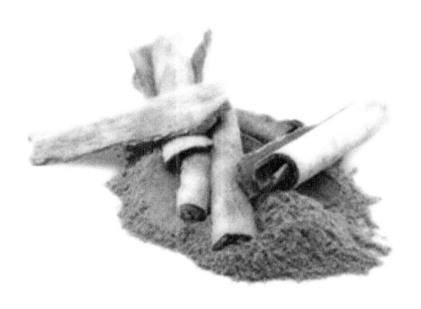

Cinnamon

Historically, cinnamon was considered more precious than gold. It is mentioned in the Bible, and was used in ancient Egypt as a beverage, in medicine, and as an embalming agent.

Cinnamon comes from the stems of the cinnamomum tree. The inner bark is extracted, and when it dries, it forms strips that curl into rolls. These are what we know as cinnamon sticks, which can then be ground into cinnamon powder.

The distinct smell and flavor of cinnamon is due to the oily compound called "cinnamaldehyde," the source of most of cinnamon's powerful effects on health and metabolism. Two other components also contribute to cinnamon's healing abilities: cinnamyl acetate, and cinnamyl alcohol, although it has a wide range of other beneficial substances.

Cinnamon is an excellent source of manganese, fiber, and calcium, and is antibacterial, antimicrobial, antifungal, antioxidant, and anti-inflammatory.

Cinnamon has been shown to be a significant contributor in treating a wide range of conditions and diseases from toenail fungus to Alzheimer's disease.

There are two types of spices that we commonly call cinnamon. Ceylon cinnamon has low levels of coumarin (0.04 percent) compared to cassia cinnamon (4 percent), which is ordinarily found at the grocery store.

It's important to keep in mind that coumarin in high doses can cause liver damage, although recent research has shown that this potentially toxic compound in cassia cinnamon bark is found primarily in the fat soluble components, while present at very low levels in water soluble cinnamon extracts. Get Ceylon cinnamon when you can, which probably calls for a trip to the health food store, or Asian marketplace.

Cinnamon as a Natural Remedy

Cinnamon is a natural remedy for many ailments – let's take a look at a few of its numerous uses:

Some people consider cinnamon to be the very best cure for stomach flu. Cinnamon is one of the most effective substances against e-coli, salmonella, and adenovirus.

Cinnamon has been used to provide relief from the common cold, mixed in a tea with some fresh ginger.

Cinnamon dramatically reduces the symptoms of IBS, especially bloating and its discomfort, by killing bacteria and healing the infections in the GI tract, which allows the gastric juices to work normally, providing relief from constipation and diarrhea.

Cinnamon has proven to stop medication-resistant candida yeast infections, and has excellent anti-microbial activity against staph infections, penicillium digitatum that can cause pneumonia, and listeria-bacteria, which causes food poisoning.

Cinnamon leaf oil is a powerful antibacterial and makes a great natural disinfectant. Dilute with water to disinfect kitchen counter tops, sinks, the refrigerator, garbage cans, door knobs, every surface in the bathroom, toys, the interior of vehicles, so forth and so on.

Cinnamon leaf oil smells great and is an effective odor neutralizer, killing bacteria that create bad odors, not just masking the odors. Two to five drops of cinnamon leaf oil mixed with water then sprayed in a diffuser, neutralizes all odors. It is more effective, less expensive and healthier than chemical sprays.

Cinnamon bark oil is also an extremely powerful antibacterial. Boil a couple of cinnamon sticks in hot water for a mild, disinfecting, face wash.

The aroma of cinnamon also has the benefit of improving your mood, especially effective during the long winter days when seasonal affective disorder (SAD) may set in.

Cinnamon also has the effect of keeping us more alert and decreases frustration when driving.

The Antimicrobial, Antibacterial, Antioxidant Activity of Cinnamon

Cinnamon's antimicrobial properties are so effective that the addition of just a few drops of cinnamon essential oil to approximately 3 ounces of refrigerated carrot broth inhibited the growth of the food borne pathogenic Bacillus cereus *for 60 days.*

When the broth was refrigerated without the addition of cinnamon oil, the pathogenic Bacillus cereus flourished. What's more, the addition of cinnamon improved the flavor of the broth.

Even more impressive, Ceylon cinnamon, in combination with turmeric and chili, preserves food without a refrigerator.

Use Cinnamon Oil coated paper as a preservative. A six percent cinnamon oil solution food packaging completely inhibited mold in sliced bread. It's also effective as an insect resistant food packaging.

Cinnamon is so powerful an antioxidant that when compared to five other antioxidant spices – anise, ginger, licorice, nutmeg and vanilla – and the chemical food preservatives, BHA (butylated hydroxyanisole), BHT (butylated hydroxytoluene), and propyl gallate, *cinnamon prevented oxidation more effectively than all the other spices and the chemical antioxidants!*

Cinnamon is a warming agent, and when combined with a carrier oil it is highly effective in relaxing and relieving muscle pain. It's great in massage therapy, or put a few drops in the bath to relax and to sooth tired and aching muscles.

You can use cinnamon sticks, tea, or powder for treatment of toenail fungus or athletes foot *internally*, and a few drops of cinnamon leaf oil in warm water *externally*, for a relaxing, healing foot soak.

Cinnamon is one of the world's top seven antioxidants. Antioxidants reduce formation of free radicals that cause cancer and many other diseases.

The antibacterial and antimicrobial properties of cinnamon will get rid of harmful bacteria in the mouth without damaging teeth or gums, preventing tooth decay and reducing bad breath. These are the reasons why cinnamon is often used in chewing gums, mouthwashes, toothpaste and breath mints.

Cinnamaldehyde, the main active component of cinnamon, helps fight various kinds of infection, effectively treating respiratory tract infections caused by fungi, while also inhibiting the growth of various bacteria.

The antimicrobial qualities of cinnamon can be used for treating and controlling head lice, black ants, bed bugs, dust mites, and roaches, and is a powerful defense against mosquitoes, killing larvae and acting as a bug repellant.

Immediately upon perceiving a sore throat or cough, brew some cinnamon tea. It's claimed that cinnamon tea will stop a cold, cough, or sore throat in its tracks, because of its antibacterial and warming properties, and its propensity to increase blood flow and improve blood oxygen levels.

Chinese medicine recommends cinnamon for phlegm coughs.

Cinnamaldehyde has been thoroughly researched for its effects on blood platelets, which are meant to clump together under emergency circumstances such as an injury, as a way to stop bleeding, but under normal circumstances, platelets can make blood flow inadequate if they clump together too much. Cinnaldehyde helps prevent unwanted clumping of blood platelets.

Because of its high levels of manganese, cinnamon may be an excellent candidate to mitigate the effects of PMS. Women with 5.6 mg of manganese in their diets each day had fewer mood swings and cramps compared to those who consumed only 1 mg of manganese.

Another clinical study found that 46 patients with PMS had significantly lower amounts of calcium, chromium, copper, and manganese in their blood.

There is supporting evidence that certain types of gut bacteria contributes to making people susceptible to depression. Cinnamon is a powerful stomach antibacterial and may help to remove bad bacteria.

However, as cinnamon removes both bad and good bacteria from the stomach it's advised to repopulate with a probiotic or eating fermented food. Which is a good idea in any case!

Cinnamon in Research
Diabetes

Cinnamon has been shown to prevent, and even, apparently, cure, diabetes. Insulin and cinnamon help cells let nutrition in and wastes out.

Insulin is essential for the transport of blood sugar from the bloodstream and into cells, but many people are resistant to the effects of insulin, resulting in serious conditions like metabolic syndrome and type 2 diabetes. Cinnamon dramatically reduces insulin resistance, thus lowering blood sugar levels.

Cinnamon decreases the amount of glucose that enters the bloodstream after a meal by interfering with the digestive enzymes, slowing the breakdown of carbohydrates in the digestive tract.

Both test tube and animal studies have shown that compounds in cinnamon stimulate insulin receptors, while inhibiting an enzyme that inactivates insulin receptors, significantly increasing the cells' ability to use glucose.

Cinnamon reduces levels of LDL cholesterol and triglycerides, while HDL cholesterol remains stable.

Numerous studies have confirmed the anti-diabetic effects of cinnamon, lowering fasting blood sugar levels 10-29 percent.

Research has shown that the insulin-enhancing complexes in cinnamon increase the body's ability to use glucose 20-fold.

A study evaluated 30 men and 30 women with type 2 diabetes, divided into six groups. Groups 1, 2, and 3 were given 1, 3, or 6 grams of cinnamon daily, Groups 4, 5, and 6 received 1, 3 or 6 grams of placebo.

Even the lowest amount of cinnamon, 1 gram per day, produced an *18 percent drop in blood sugar*. Cholesterol and triglycerides were lowered as well. When daily cinnamon was stopped, blood sugar levels began to increase.

After 40 days, all three levels of administered cinnamon reduced blood sugar levels by 18-29 percent, triglycerides reduced 23-30 percent, LDL cholesterol reduced 7-27 percent, and total cholesterol reduced 12-26 percent. No significant changes were seen in the groups receiving a placebo.

When rats were given a daily dose of cinnamon at 300 mg per kilogram of body weight for a three week period, their skeletal muscle absorbed 17 percent more blood sugar per minute compared to that of control rats, which had not received cinnamon.

Seasoning a high carb food with cinnamon can help lessen its impact on your blood sugar levels. Cinnamon slows the rate at which the stomach empties after meals, reducing the rise in blood sugar after eating.

At the same time, these various factors drastically cut the risk of heart disease.

Cinnamon's Calcium and Fiber

In addition to its unique essential oils, cinnamon is an excellent source of fiber, manganese and calcium. The combination of calcium and fiber in cinnamon is important because they bind to bile salts, which assists in removing them from the body.

Removing bile prevents the damage bile salts can cause to colon cells, thus reducing the risk of colon cancer. And when bile is removed by fiber, the body breaks down cholesterol to make new bile, lowering high cholesterol levels. This, of course, helps prevent atherosclerosis and heart disease.

Cinnamon oil is a promising solution in the treatment of tumors, gastric cancers, melanomas, leukemia and lymphoma cancer cells. Research has shown that sugar may be causing, or at least sustaining, cancer cells. Cinnamon has a mitigating effect by controlling blood sugar levels in the body.

Cinnamon reduces the growth of cancer cells and the formation of blood vessels in tumors. Like turmeric and ginger, it appears to be toxic to cancer cells, causing cell death.

In a study of mice with colon cancer, cinnamon was a potent activator of detoxifying enzymes in the colon, protecting against further cancer growth.

Cinnamon's two chemical constituents, cinnamaldehyde and eugenol, have been used to develop nutraceuticals effective in fighting human colon cancer cells with eugenol, and human hepatoma cells with cinnamaldehyde. Cinnamon starves cancer cells of the sugar needed to sustain them.

Cinnamon has high levels of manganese – 73 percent of daily minimum requirement in two sticks of cinnamon. The body needs manganese for optimal bone health as it is used to build bones, blood, and other connective tissues. People who are deficient in the mineral are more likely to develop osteoporosis.

Alzheimer's Disease

The neurodegenerative diseases, Alzheimer's and Parkinson's, are characterized by the progressive loss of the structure and function of brain cells.

The latest findings indicate that two compounds found in cinnamon—cinnamaldehyde and epicatechin—are effective in fighting Alzheimer's, inhibiting the buildup of the protein tau in the brain.

Cinnamon has also been shown to prevent the development of the filamentous "tangles" found in the brain cells that characterize Alzheimer's, while an Israeli study concluded that cinnamon can delay the effects of five aggressive strains of Alzheimer's inducing genes.

Orally administered cinnamon extract has been successful in correcting cognitive impairment in animals with Alzheimer's disease.

Parkinson's Disease

Rush University Medical Center found that using cinnamon can reverse the cellular, biomechanical, and anatomical changes that occur in the brains of mice with Parkinson's disease.

In a study of mice with Parkinson's disease, cinnamon helped to protect neurons, normalize neurotransmitter levels, and improve motor function.

Cinnamon's Antiviral Effect

HIV is a virus that slowly breaks down the immune system, which can eventually lead to AIDS if untreated. A Cinnamon derived procyanidin polymer extracted from cassia varieties of cinnamon helps fight against HIV-1, the most common strain of the HIV virus in humans.

A laboratory study looking at HIV infected cells found that cinnamon was the most effective treatment of all 69 medicinal plants studied.

Eugenol is effective against the virus, herpes.

Cinnamaldehye is effective against the adenovirus, an infection that is the most common cause of illness in the respiratory system.

Just smelling cinnamon boosts brain activity! Research found that chewing cinnamon flavored gum or simply smelling cinnamon, enhanced study participants' cognitive processing, improving scores on attention-demanding tasks, working memory, virtual recognition memory, and visual-motor speed.

Participants were exposed to four conditions: no odor, peppermint, jasmine, or cinnamon, with cinnamon emerging the clear winner in producing positive effects on brain function.

An Ounce of Prevention

In humans with type 2 diabetes, consuming as little as 1 gram of cinnamon per day reduces blood sugar, triglycerides, and LDL (bad) cholesterol.

If you have stomach cramps or upsets, a cup of cinnamon tea two-to-three times per day will reduce the pain, gas, and bloating.

The effective dose for diabetics or to prevent diabetes is one-to-six grams of cinnamon per day (0.5-2 teaspoons).

How to Select and Store Cinnamon

Cinnamon is available in stick or powder form. While the sticks can be stored for longer, the ground powder has a stronger flavor. If possible, smell the cinnamon to make sure that it has a sweet smell, which indicates that it is fresh.

Keep cinnamon in a tightly sealed glass container in a cool, dark and dry place. Ground cinnamon will keep for about six months, while cinnamon sticks will stay fresh for about one year stored this way. Or store in the refrigerator to extend its freshness even longer. If the cinnamon does not smell sweet, it is no longer fresh.

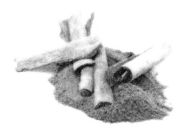

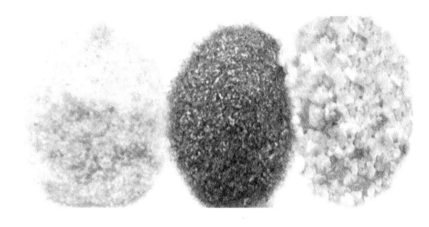

Sea Salt

The Greek philosopher Pythagorus said that salt is born of the purest parents, the sun and the sea. Salt has its origin in the sea, whether taken directly from the sea, or taken from deposits created eons ago by the ocean and salty streams that once flowed through caves. There are many kinds of sea salt from all around the world.

Sea Salt and pH Balance

Sea salt provides good skin care, improves dental health, offers relief from rheumatoid arthritis, muscle cramps, psoriasis, osteoarthritis, acne and rhino-sinusitis, it's beneficial for exfoliation, and as a nasal and eye wash.

Sea salt helps to keep the body alkaline, in perfect pH balance by flushing excess acids. When the pH value of the blood moves toward acidic, it disturbs the healthy balance of the body, resulting in chronic and serious medical conditions.

Keeping your body's pH in balance regulates your heart beat, allows for a great night's sleep, neutralizes disease process, all while keeping you energized and mentally sharp. (To learn more about pH balance, read *How to Save Your Life with the Power of pH Balance*.)

The wide array of colors of sea salt is due to the absorption of minerals from the earth that line the body of water.

Regular, homogenous, white table salt has been iodized – which contributes to high blood pressure, bleached and diluted, with other chemicals added as well, stealing the beneficial minerals and elements from the salt.

Preparation of sea salt includes very little processing, allowing it to retain its treasure of elements and minerals. Furthermore, the form of these minerals and elements are readily absorbed by the human body.

Celtic sea salt, slightly moist and flecked with gray minerals, is harvested entirely by hand with only the use of wooden tools. It just doesn't get more natural than that!

Sea salt can have up to 82 nutrients, including, but clearly not limited to: sodium, calcium, bromide, chloride, copper, iron, magnesium, potassium, and zinc.

Sea Salt as a Natural Remedy

Salt and potassium provide improved electrolytic balance of the body, which is necessary to every cellular function. There are so many ways sea salt can improve your health. Let's look at a few.

Skin & Skeleton

For skin care, the mineral content in Dead Sea salt is appreciated for the rejuvenating effects on the skin. Bathing in a Dead Sea salt solution helps keep the skin revitalized and moisturized. Dead Sea salt baths also eliminate the roughness and inflammation on the skin's surface.

Exfoliation with sea salts removes dead skin, tones up skin tissues, and stimulates peripheral blood circulation. The granular texture of sea salt provides clean and smooth skin. Also, sea salts contain sulphur which helps in cleansing and treating skin conditions such as dermatitis and acne.

A sea salt scrub is excellent for patients with low blood pressure, epilepsy, poor blood circulation, and general fatigue, by promoting healthy blood circulation.

The anti-inflammatory effect of sea salt is due to the presence of a high magnesium content, which helps the body flush out toxins from the pores while improving blood circulation.

A bath containing sea salts has anti-inflammatory qualities and has shown significant improvements for those suffering from rheumatoid arthritis.

Twenty-five percent of the body's salt is stored in the bones helping to keep them strong. With inadequate salt, the body draws sodium from the bones, leading to osteoporosis. Always drink plenty of water and add a pinch of sea salt to help prevent osteoporosis.

Sea salt contains fluoride, which, in this natural state, is quite beneficial for dental health. Fluoride protects teeth from acidic damage and cavities. Regular rinsing and gargling with tepid sea salt water will alleviate a sore throat, bleeding gums, mouth sores, and mouth ulcers.

Sea salt assists in weight loss by helping the body create digestive juices to faster and more efficiently digest food, thus preventing buildup in the digestive tract which leads to constipation and weight gain.

Along with proper medication, treatment with sea salt has shown to be effective on psoriasis. It has also shown significant improvements in patients suffering from itching and scaling skin, hives, and skin rashes.

Further, therapeutic sea salt baths with mud packs and sulfur for psoriasis and psoriatic arthritis sufferers has promising results, including a reduction in spinal pain and increased flexibility of the spine.

Research supports notable improvements among patients with knee osteoarthritis after balneotherapy with Dead Sea salt. These improvements were sustained for several weeks.

Rhino-sinusitis responds well to Dead Sea salt treatment. Nasal irrigation with sea salt shows better relief than those made of a hypertonic saline solution.

Sea salt's anti-inflammatory properties helps to alleviate swelling and congestion, and make it a better alternative for treating nasal allergies and other respiratory disorders than nasal steroids, which can have negative side effects such as inflammation.

It's not commonly known, but I'll bet this will be one of your favorite things to learn about sea salt – it stimulates healthy hair growth. Gently massage your scalp with sea salt to improve blood circulation and to strengthen hair follicles. It's also an effective treatment for dandruff.

Sea salt will relieve muscle cramps and improve muscular strength. The therapeutic qualities of magnesium and potassium make sea salt an outstanding remedy for aches and pains. A sea salt bath prevents the buildup of toxins in the body, easing stiffness caused by muscle fatigue and tension.

Nothing feels as lovely after a long day on one's feet as a foot soak in a warm sea salt solution, relaxing muscles and relieving soreness and pain.

Diabetes & Heart Health

Sea salts helps in maintaining optimum levels of blood sugar, and is effective in reducing being dependent on insulin medication for the regulation of sugar levels.

Sea salt contributes to maintaining a healthy electrolyte balance in the body. This is necessary to maintain optimum blood circulation and composition, muscular strength, and overall bodily function. Potassium, calcium, magnesium, and sodium are important minerals to maintain the electrolytic equilibrium of the body.

Because sea salt helps to maintain healthy blood pressure, it also helps normalize irregular heartbeats, which contributes to preventing various cardiac disorders. Sea salt also helps reduce high cholesterol levels, high blood pressure and help to regulate an irregular heart beat, which contributes to preventing atherosclerosis, heart attacks and strokes.

Sea Salt's Antidepressant Effects

Calming and stress-relieving, a sea salt compress will reduce dark circles and puffiness under the eyes.

Sea salt helps preserve the body's store of serotonin and melatonin, two essential hormones that contribute to calming stress and depression. When you feel good, you are more relaxed and sleep better at night – an upward healthy spiral!

Stress & depression free = better sleep
Better sleep = stress & depression free

Nighty-night! Sea salt baths have a soporific effect, and contribute to a wonderful, rejuvenating, health-restoring sleep.

How to Select and Store Sea Salt

There are many delightful kinds of sea salt to choose from. Experiment and enjoy! Be sure to keep your sea salt in a tightly sealed container – a few grains of brown rice will help absorb moisture.

Please keep in mind that *excessive* intake of any kind of salt can lead to edema or high blood pressure. Be sure to maintain appropriate levels of salt intake.

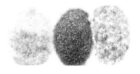

The End

I'm so glad you've read *Save Your Life with Stupendous Spices.* I trust you've discovered information you can use in your everyday life to contribute to your optimum health – which leads to optimum happiness!

Your Gift

My gift to you, from the pages of
Horn of Plenty — The Cornucopia of Your Life
download at:
bit.ly / hornofplentygift

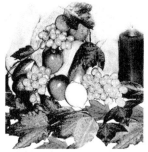

Other books in the *How to Save Your Life* series:
Save Your Life with the Power of pH Balance
Save Your Life with the phenomenal Lemon (& Lime!)
And watch for the soon-to-be-released:
Save Your Life with the Elixir of Water

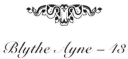

NOTE:

This content is not intended to be medical advice or instructions for medical diagnosis or treatment. Nothing in these contents should be considered to diagnose, treat, cure, or prevent disease without the supervision of a qualified healthcare provider.

About the Author

It's about You – but here's a few words about me to inspire your trust in what I write....

I know that a happy, kind, productive world evolves from happy, kind, productive, individual people.

The goal of my writing is to help clear your path to joyful productivity, in the glow of a healthy, contented, and meaningful life.

A Bitty-Bit of Bio....

I received my Doctorate from the University of California at Irvine in the School of Social Sciences, with a focus on psychology and ethnography. I've always been relentlessly curious about how people think, and how those thoughts make them feel.

After I submitted my doctoral dissertation, I moved to the Pacific Northwest, to write and to have a small private psychotherapy practice in a tiny town not much bigger than a village.

I worked with many amazing people, and witnessed astounding emotional, psychological, and spiritual, healing.

It was a wonderful experience. But after twenty plus years, I realized it was time to put my focus on my writing, wherein I could potentially help greater numbers of people. Where I could meet *you!*

I live on ten acres of forest with a few domestic and numerous wild creatures. Along with creating an ever-growing inventory of books, my writing has appeared in hundreds of online and print publications.

Your support of my writing helps support ten acres of natural forest, and all its resident fauna. *All the creatures and I thank you!*

Questions, comments, observations, reviews? I'd love to hear from you!:

Blythe@BlytheAyne.com

www.BlytheAyne.com

Printed in Great Britain
by Amazon

55991854R00030